Vegan Diet Cookbook

Satisfying Meat-Free Recipes for a Planted-Based Diet

Jessie Barnes

the reader will render any resulting actions solely under their purview. There are no scenarios in which the publisher or the original author of this work can be in any fashion deemed liable for any hardship or damages that may befall them after undertaking information described herein.

Additionally, the information in the following pages is intended only for informational purposes and should thus be thought of as universal. As befitting its nature, it is presented without assurance regarding its prolonged validity or interim quality. Trademarks that are mentioned are done without written consent and can in no way be considered an endorsement from the trademark holder.

Table of Contents

INTRODUCTION

Veganism is a way of life that tries to avoid as much as possible the use of animals in food, clothing, footwear, cosmetics, and any other aspect of life, to reduce animal suffering.

Veganism includes a 100% plant diet.

A vegan does not consume any animal product - no egg, no dairy products, and no meat of any kind." Many vegans also avoid honey and some even do not use or wear products made with animal fur, skin, bones, etc...

There are many vegan substitutes for eggs and dairy products.

Healthy vegans eat a wide variety of foods to ensure they get all the necessary nutrients that their body needs, such as vitamin 8-12, iron, and proteins. There are lots of sources of these nutrients in the vegan diet. It is just a myth that vegans suffer nutritional deficiencies. The vegan diet has tremendous health benefits as well. Not only can it prevent diseases such as cancer, type II diabetes, arthritis, osteoporosis, obesity, heart diseases, and more.

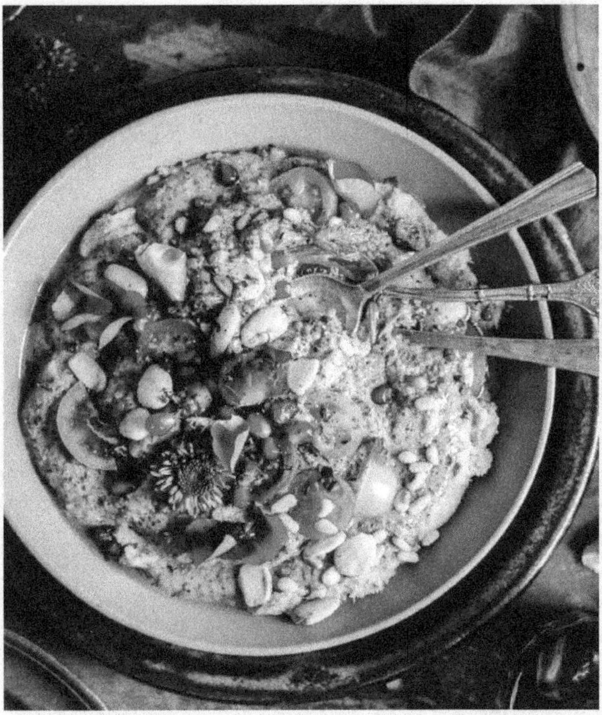

Vegan Recipes

Sunrise Smoothie

5 minutes

0 minutes

4 Servings

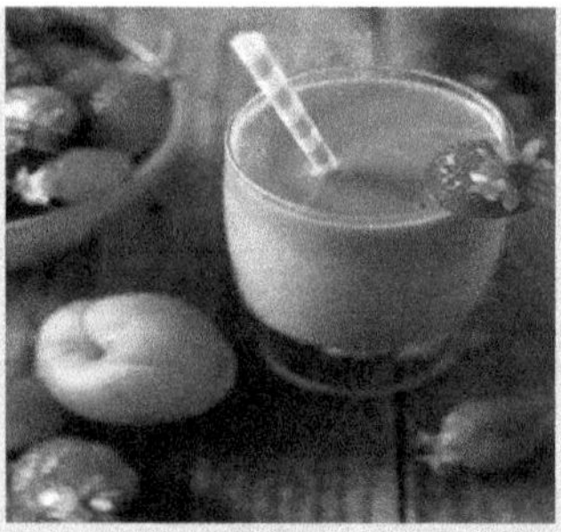

INGREDIENTS

- 4 tablespoons chia seed
- 2 frozen banana
- 2 lemon, peeled
- 2 cups diced carrots
- 4 clementine, peeled
- 4 cups frozen strawberries, unsweetened
- 12 tablespoons pomegranate tendrils
- 2 cup almond milk, unsweetened

COOKING STEPS

1. Add all the ingredients in the order into a food processor or blender and then pulse for 1 to 2 minutes until blended, scraping the sides of the container frequently.
2. Distribute the smoothie among glasses and then serve.

ORANGE FRENCH TOAST

5 minutes | 30 minutes | 8 Servings

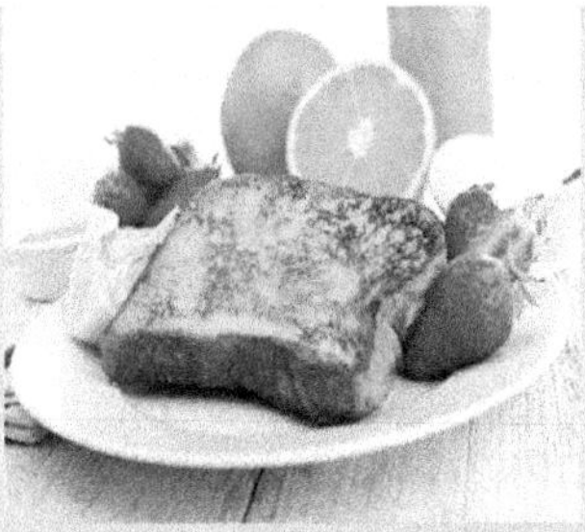

INGREDIENTS

- 2 cups of plant milk (unflavored)
- Four tablespoon maple syrup
- 11/2 tablespoon cinnamon
- Salt (optional)
- 1 cup flour (almond)
- 1 tablespoon orange zest
- 8 bread slices

COOKING STEPS

1. Turn the oven and heat to 400 degrees F afterward.
2. In a cup, add Ingredients: and whisk until the batter is smooth.
3. Dip each piece of bread into the paste and permit to soak for a couple of seconds.
4. Put in the pan, and cook until lightly browned.
5. Put the toast on the cookie sheet and bake for ten to fifteen minutes in the oven, until it is crispy.

Mustard Sauce

15 minutes

10 minutes

4 Servings

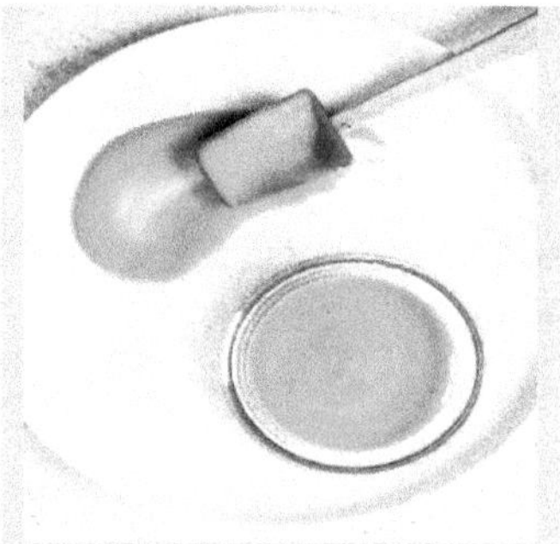

INGREDIENTS

- 30 g margarine
- 30 grams of flour
- 500 ml vegetable broth
- 2 tbsp mustard
- Lemon juice
- Salt and sugar

COOKING STEPS

1. First, heat the margarine in a saucepan and melt it. Then stir in the flour with a whisk so that there are no more lumps in it.
2. Then deglaze the sauce with the vegetable stock and season with salt, sugar, and lemon juice.

Rice Pancakes

10 minutes

10 minutes

4 Servings

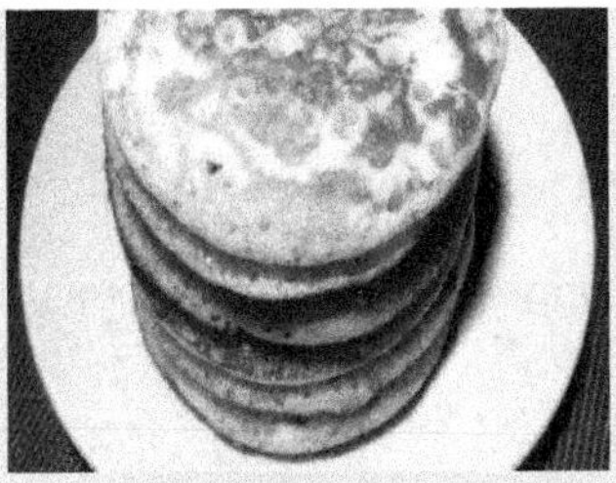

INGREDIENTS

- 100g of rice flour
- 150ml of rice milk
- 1 tablespoon Sunflower or coconut oil (to your liking)
- 1 tablespoon Flax seeds soaked 15 min in 3 tablespoons of Water (to replace the egg)
- 1 pic. of salt

COOKING STEPS

1. Add the flour, salt, milk, and oil to a bowl and beat with a whisk.
2. Then add the flaxseed and blend well into the preparation.
3. Let stand an hour in the refrigerator.
4. Remove and spoon the batter into a hot, greased skillet.
5. Leave them for a few minutes on each side and place on a large plate until cool.

Super-Fruit Bowl

10 minutes | 0 minutes | 2 Servings

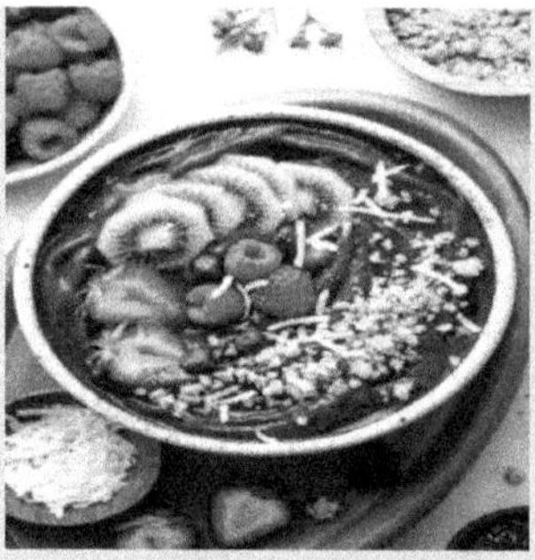

Ingredients

- Kiwi
- 4 tablespoons of chia
- 100 g of blackberries
- 100 g raspberries
- 100 g blackberries
- 100 g pineapple
- 50 g of grated coconut
- 12 almonds
- 100 g of yogurt (vegan) of blackberries (or your preference)

Cooking Steps

1. Peel and cut the kiwi into slices and wash all the red fruits.
2. Add all the ingredients harmoniously in a bowl and at the end add a portion of the blackberry yogurt.

SWEET CREPES

5 minutes

8 minutes

5 Servings

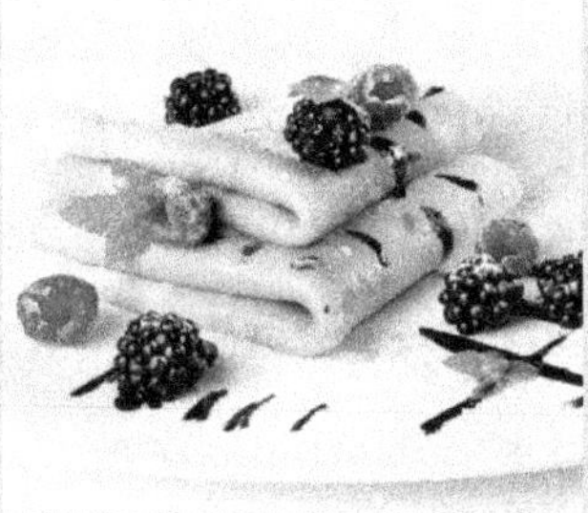

INGREDIENTS

- 1 cup of water
- 1 banana
- 1/2 cup oat flour
- 1/2 cup brown rice flour
- 1 teaspoon baking powder
- 1 tablespoon coconut sugar
- 1/8 teaspoon salt

COOKING STEPS

1. Take a blender, place all the ingredients in it except for sugar and salt, and pulse for 1 minute until smooth.
2. Take a skillet pan, place it over medium-high heat, grease it with oil, and when hot, pour in ¼ cup of batter, spread it as thin as possible, then cook for few minutes per side until golden brown.
3. Sprinkle with sugar and serve.

HERB AND CHEESE OMELET

5 minutes | 5 minutes | 2 Servings

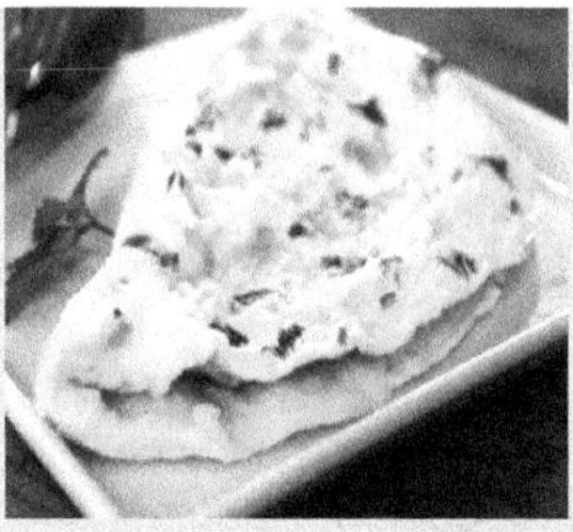

INGREDIENTS

- 4 eggs Salt and pepper to taste
- 2 tbsp. low-fat milk
- 1 tsp. chives, chopped
- 1 tbsp. parsley, chopped ½
- cup goat cheese crumbled
- 1 tsp. olive oil

COOKING STEPS

1. Beat the eggs in a bowl. Stir in the salt, pepper, and milk. In a bowl, combine the chives, parsley, and goat cheese, then pour the oil into a pan over medium heat.
2. Cook the eggs for 3 minutes. Add the cheese mixture on top.
3. Fold and serve.

SWEET POMEGRANATE PORRIDGE

5 minutes

30 minutes

4 Servings

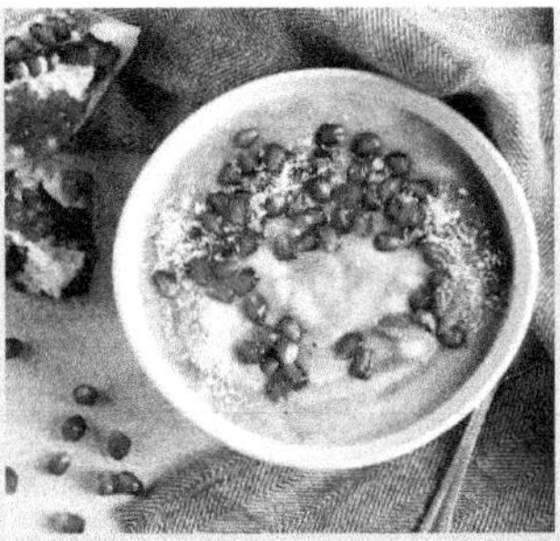

INGREDIENTS

- 2 Cups Oats
- 1 ½ Cups Water
- 1 ½ Cups Pomegranate Juice
- 2 Tablespoons Pomegranate Molasses

COOKING STEPS

1. Pour all ingredients into the instant pot and mix well.
2. Cook on high pressure for four minutes.
3. Use a quick release, and serve warm.

GUACAMOLE ON BREAD WITH SMOKED TOFU

5 minutes | 5 minutes | 2 Servings

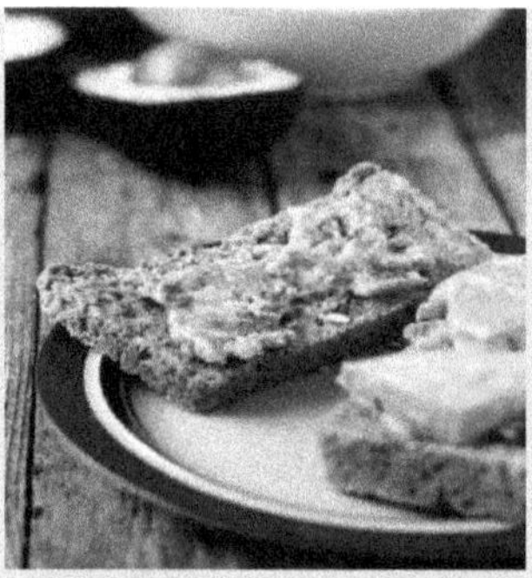

INGREDIENTS

- 1 ripe avocado
- 1 medium tomato
- 1 onion
- 4 slices of whole-grain bread
- The juice of half a lemon
- Salt, pepper, chili to taste
- 100 g smoked tofu

COOKING STEPS

1. First scrape out the pulp of the avocado, mash it with a fork, and then cut the tomato and onion into small pieces.
2. Mix everything together and season with lemon juice, salt, pepper, and chili and spread on the wholemeal bread.
3. Cut the smoked tofu into slices and fry briefly on both sides.
4. Divide and serve the bread.

Classic Bircher Muesli

15 minutes | 0 minutes | 1 Servings

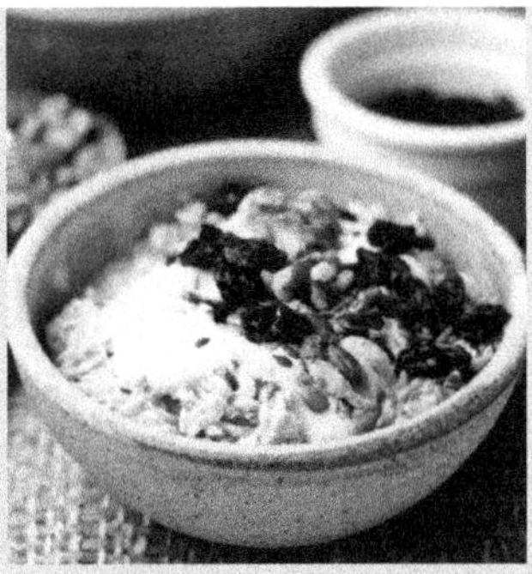

INGREDIENTS

- 4 tablespoons of oatmeal
- 150 ml almond milk
- 1 red apple
- 1 tbsp chopped nuts of your choice (e.g. macadamia or hazelnuts)
- 1 teaspoon agave syrup

COOKING STEPS

1. Put the oat flakes and almond milk in a bowl, stir and place in the refrigerator overnight.
2. Wash and core the red apple and cut it into small cubes.
3. Then add the nuts, apple, and agave syrup to the oat flakes, stir and enjoy.

Chocolate Peanut Bowl

15 minutes | 10 minutes | 2 Servings

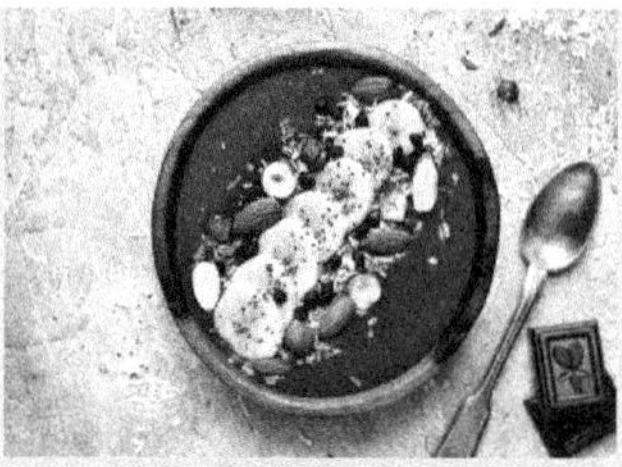

Ingredients

- 100 g oat flakes, tender
- 250 ml of plant milk
- 2 tbsp peanut butter
- 1 banana
- 1 teaspoon cocoa powder, raw
- 30 grams of salted peanuts
- 30 g dark chocolate

Cooking Steps

1. First heat the vegetable milk in a saucepan and then stir in the oat flakes, peanut butter, and cocoa powder. Remove from heat and let soak for 5 minutes before dividing the porridge into two bowls.
2. Chop the peanuts just like the chocolate and cut the banana into very fine slices.
3. Then distribute these ingredients decoratively as a topping on the oatmeal mixture.

Breakfast Scramble

10 minutes | 30 minutes | 6 Servings

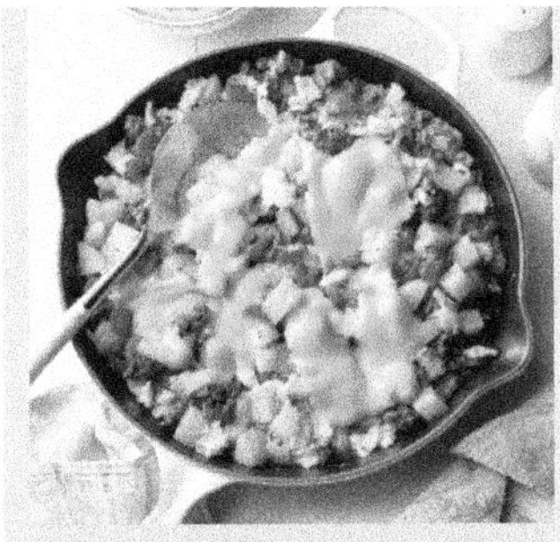

INGREDIENTS

- 1 red onion
- 1 to 2 tablespoons soy sauce
- 2 cups sliced mushrooms
- Salt to taste
- 1 1/2 teaspoon black pepper
- 1 1/2 teaspoons turmeric
- 1/4 teaspoon cayenne
- 3 cloves garlic
- 1 red bell pepper

COOKING STEPS

1. In a small pan, put all vegetables and cook until crispy.
2. Stir in the cauliflower and cook for four to six minutes or until it smooth.
3. Add spices to the pan and cook for another five minutes.

- 1 large head cauliflower
- 1 green bell pepper

Vegan Breakfast Biscuits

10 minutes

10 minutes

6 Servings

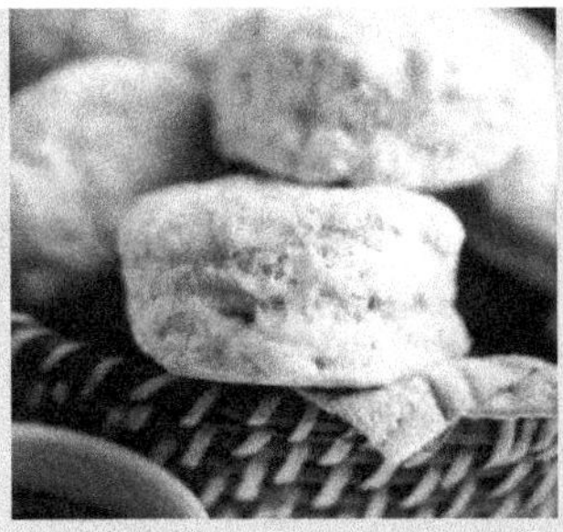

INGREDIENTS

- cups Almond Flour
- 1 tbsp. Baking Powder
- ¼ teaspoon Salt
- ½ teaspoon Onion Powder
- ½ cup Coconut Milk
- ¼ cup Nutritional Yeast
- 2 tbsp. Ground Flax Seeds
- ¼ cup Olive Oil

COOKING STEPS

1. Preheat oven to 450F.
2. Whisk together all ingredients in a bowl.
3. Divide the batter into a pre-greased muffin tin.
4. Bake for 10 minutes.

Chayote Fricassee

15 minutes | 15 minutes | 3 Servings

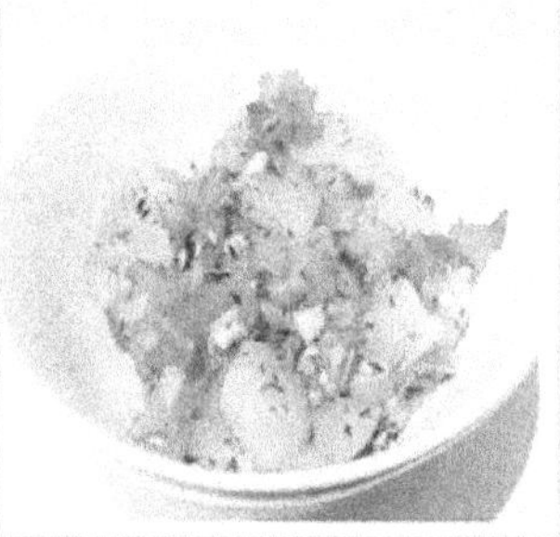

Ingredients

- 1 kg of chayote
- 4 tomatoes, small
- 1 clove of garlic
- 2 onions
- 1 piece of ginger, small
- 200 ml of water
- 100 ml of oil
- 1 tbsp thyme, dried
- 3 tbsp parsley
- salt and pepper

Cooking Steps

1. First, wash the chayote fruits, cut them into quarters, and remove the core and core. Then peel the fruit and cut it into ½ cm thick slices. Peel the onions and garlic and cut the onions into rings and finely grate the garlic and ginger.
2. Mash the onion vegetables and ginger with a little salt in a mortar and wash the tomatoes, remove the greens and finely dice them.
3. Now heat the oil in a saucepan and briefly fry the onions and tomatoes in it. Add the chayote and stir everything. Fry the whole thing for about 5 minutes and then add the garlic and ginger.
4. Season with salt, pepper, and thyme. Deglaze with water and let the dish simmer for around 20 minutes.
5. Garnish with fresh parsley to serve.

Cauliflower Cream and Coconut Milk

10 minutes

10 minutes

2 Servings

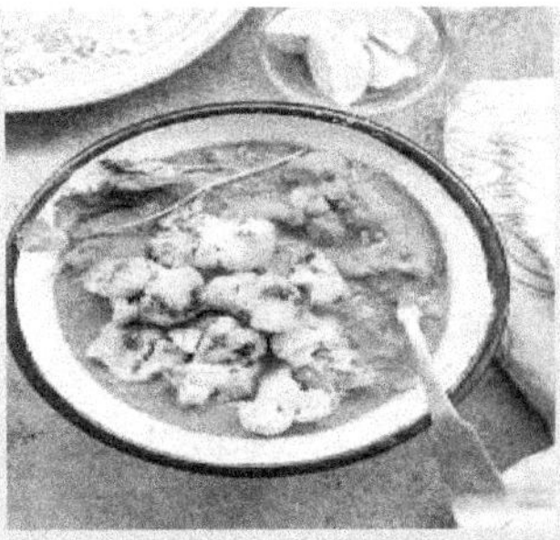

INGREDIENTS

- 1 small cooked eggplant
- 1 cup of cooked cauliflower
- 100 ml of coconut milk or cream
- Salt and pepper to taste
- Brewer's yeast and seeds for garnish (optional)

COOKING STEPS

1. Add the cooked and diced aubergine, cauliflower, coconut milk, curry, salt, and pepper to the blender.
2. Process well until a homogeneous cream consistency is achieved.
3. Serve in a bowl and garnish with brewer's yeast and seeds.

Veggie Sandwich

10 minutes | 5 minutes | 1 Servings

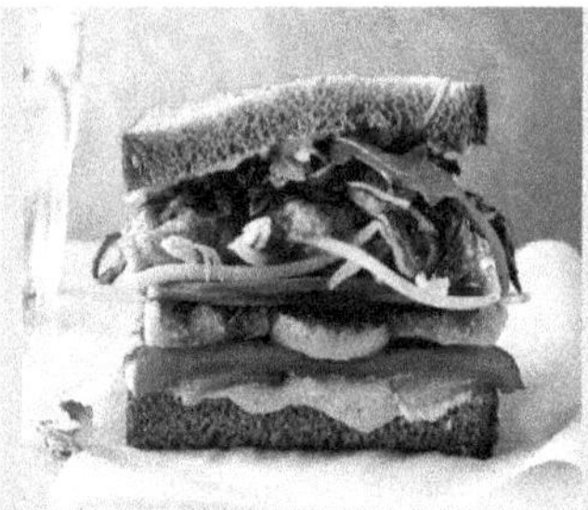

INGREDIENTS

- Whole Wheat Sandwich Bread
- Hummus (of your preference)
- Spinach sprouts
- ½ carrot
- 1 radish
- Broccoli sprouts
- Sesame seeds
- Extra virgin olive oil

COOKING STEPS

1. First, we have to prepare the hummus.
2. You can toast the bread or take it as is.
3. Spread the hummus on both slices and sprinkle with sesame seeds. Add the spinach sprouts, the carrot, and the radishes cut into slices with the help of a peeler, broccoli sprouts, and add a drizzle of oil to make it juicier.

Chickpeas Curry

10 minutes | 15 minutes | 2 Servings

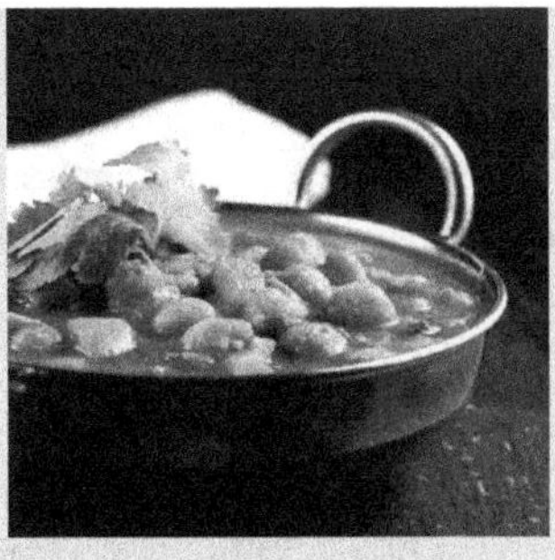

INGREDIENTS

- A can of cooked chickpeas
- 4 tablespoons oil
- Salt
- Spices: curry, cumin, pepper, paprika, and turmeric

COOKING STEPS

1. Add the chickpeas to a bowl.
2. Add a teaspoon of each of the spices (curry, paprika, cumin, and turmeric), salt, and oil.
3. Mix well.
4. Pour the chickpeas on a baking sheet and bake at 200 ° for about 15 minutes.

Black Beans and Rice

10 minutes | 30 minutes | 4 Servings

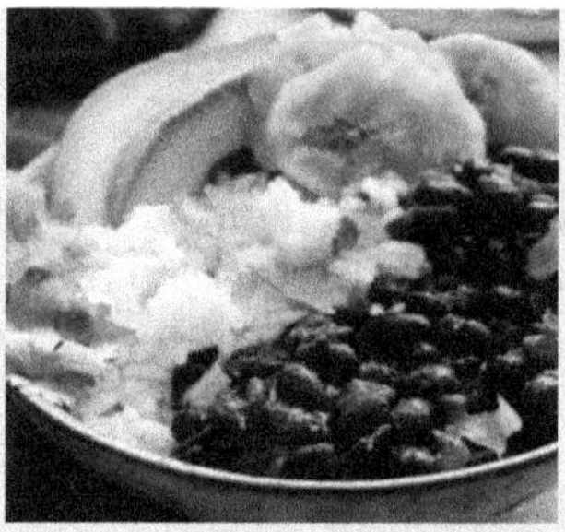

INGREDIENTS

- 3/4 cup white rice
- 1 medium white onion, peeled, chopped
- 3 1/2 cups cooked black beans
- 1 teaspoon minced garlic
- 1/4 teaspoon cayenne pepper
- 1 teaspoon ground cumin
- 1 teaspoon olive oil
- 1 1/2 cups vegetable broth

COOKING STEPS

1. Take a large pot over medium-high heat, add oil and when hot, add onion and garlic and cook for 4 minutes until saute. Then stir in rice, cook for 2 minutes, pour in the broth, bring it to a boil, switch heat to the low level and cook for 20 minutes until tender.
2. Stir in remaining ingredients, cook for 2 minutes, and then serve straight away.

QUINOA AND CHICKPEAS SALAD

10 minutes | 0 minutes | 4 Servings

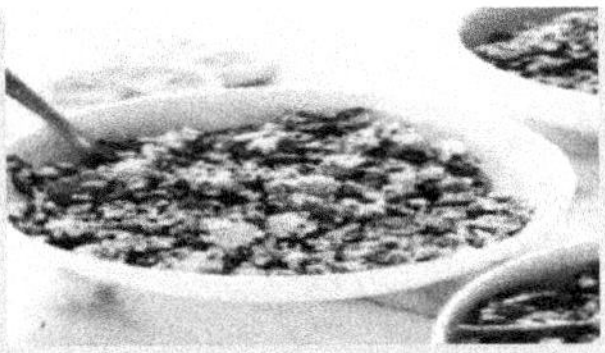

INGREDIENTS

- 3/4 cup chopped broccoli
- 1/2 cup quinoa, cooked
- 15 ounces cooked chickpeas
- ½ teaspoon minced garlic
- 1/3 teaspoon ground black pepper
- 2/3 teaspoon salt
- 1 teaspoon dried tarragon
- 2 teaspoons mustard
- 1 tablespoon lemon juice
- 3 tablespoons olive oil

COOKING STEPS

1. Take a large bowl, place all the ingredients in it, and stir until well combined.
2. Serve straight away.

EASY MEAN WHITE BEAN DIP

10 minutes | 30 minutes | 10 Servings

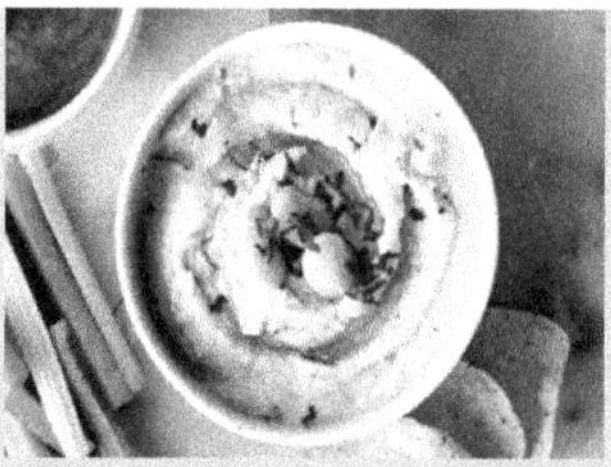

INGREDIENTS

- 3 minced garlic cloves
- 16 ounces white beans
- 1 tbsp. olive oil
- 2 tbsp. lemon juice
- 1 tsp. salt
- ½ tsp. cumin
- 1 tsp. chili powder
- 3 drops hot pepper sauce

COOKING STEPS

1. Place all the ingredients together in a food processor, and process them for about two minutes or until they're smooth.
2. If your mixture is too thick and chunky, add water to the food processor until you reach your desired consistency.
3. Enjoy!

Crunchy Fennel From The Grill

10 minutes | 10 minutes | 2 Servings

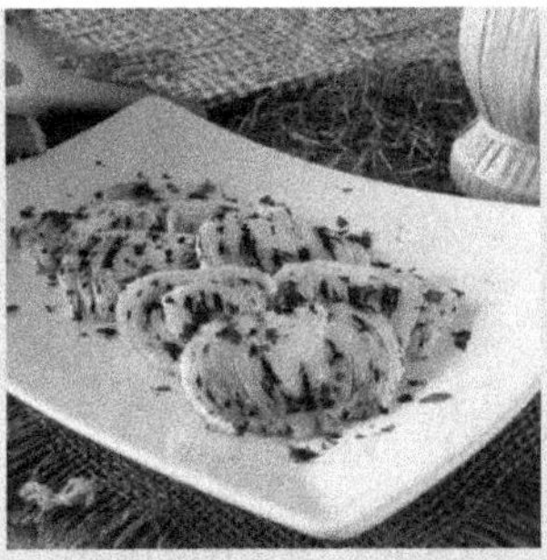

INGREDIENTS

- 2 large fennel bulbs
- 10 grams of olive oil
- ½ sprig of fresh rosemary
- Salt and pepper as needed

COOKING STEPS

1. Wash the fennel under clean water and remove the outer parts if necessary.
2. Now cut the tubers lengthways into slices and grill them on the grillage for about 3 minutes on each side.
3. While the fennel slices are roasting on the grill, the rosemary is washed under clear water, dried, and pulled from the stem.
4. Place the rosemary between the grilled fennel slices and drizzle with olive oil. Season to taste with salt and pepper before enjoying.

Creamy Aubergines with Crisp, Fruity Pomegranate Seeds

10 minutes | 25 minutes | 4 Servings

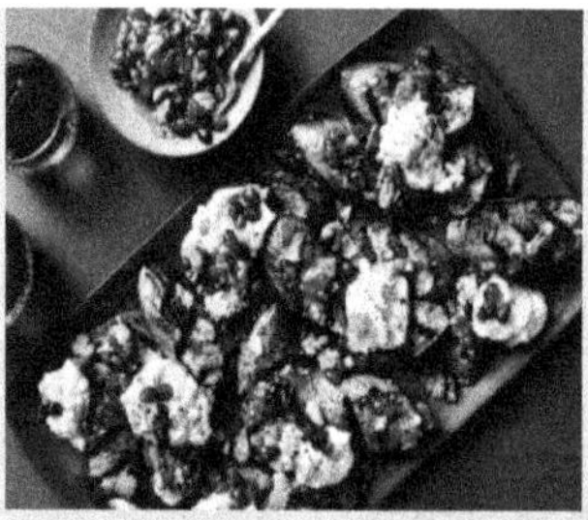

Ingredients

- 2 large eggplants
- 1 small pomegranate
- ½ bunch of fresh parsley
- 1 small clove of garlic
- 20 grams of olive oil
- 5 grams of balsamic vinegar
- Salt and pepper as needed

Cooking Steps

1. Wash the aubergines with clear, cold water, remove the stem and then cut in half lengthways. Spread salt on the side of the cut surface and let the aubergine halves steep for about 10 minutes while the rest of the ingredients are prepared. Halve the pomegranate and remove the stones from the fruit.
2. Wash the parsley under clear, cold water, pluck the leaves from the stem, dry, and then finely chop with a sharp knife.
3. Remove the garlic from its skin, finely chop it and mix it with 15 grams of olive oil in a bowl.
4. Pat the aubergines dry before brushing them with half of the garlic oil and grilling on the grill for about 12 minutes. During the grilling process, the aubergines are repeatedly coated with garlic oil.
5. Arrange the finished aubergines on a plate and serve with the pomegranate seeds and chopped parsley. Season to taste with sea salt and finally drizzle with balsamic vinegar.

HEARTY LARGE GRILLED MUSHROOMS

10 minutes	10 minutes	4 Servings

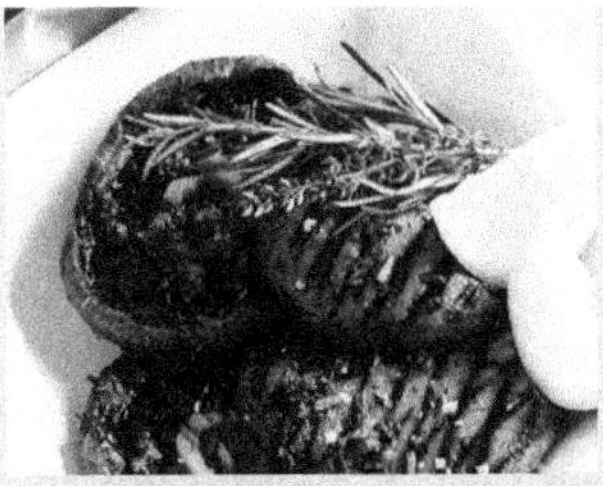

INGREDIENTS

- 250 grams of portobello edible mushrooms
- 20 grams of olive oil
- 1 two fresh rosemary
- Salt and pepper as needed

COOKING STEPS

1. Clean the mushrooms well and thoroughly with the help of a kitchen towel and remove dirt and grime.
2. Wash the rosemary under fresh, clear water, and then remove it from the stem.
3. Mix them together with the oil and rosemary in a bowl and then either place them on the grill or put them in an ovenproof dish.
4. Grill the mushrooms for about 10 minutes and then season with salt and pepper as required and to taste.

HEALTHY VEGAN BURGERS

40 minutes

40 minutes

2 Servings

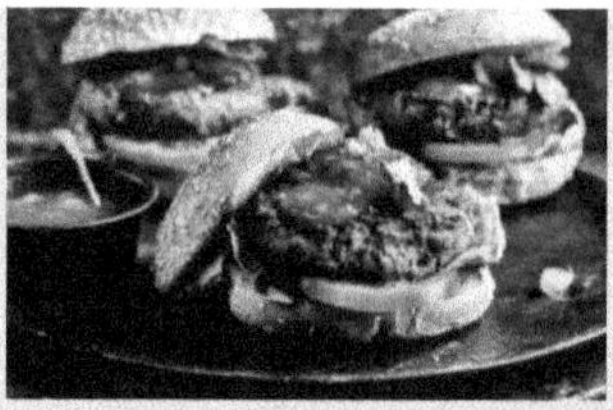

INGREDIENTS

- 200 g potatoes, if possible floury
- 100 g carrots
- 1 tbsp soy flour
- 1 tbsp rapeseed oil
- salt, pepper

For the burger:

- 2 bread rolls, whole grain
- 3 large lettuce leaves
- 1 large tomato
- Chives, cut into small rolls
- 100 g soy yogurt, unsweetened

COOKING STEPS

1. First, the vegan patties are prepared, which are considered to be a meatball substitute.
2. The potatoes are peeled and cooked for 20 minutes in boiling salted water. Cut the carrot into cubes and add to the potatoes after 15 minutes. Then mash both with a fork or a potato masher to puree.
3. The flour is stirred into the potato and carrot mixture, which should then be strongly seasoned with salt and pepper. Shape this mixture into two round patties reminiscent of meatballs and fry them on both sides in the oil in a pan.
4. Mix the soy yogurt with the chives in a bowl and season with salt and pepper. The rolls are now cut open and served with soy yogurt, lettuce leaves, tomato slices, and the pattie. Fold up the burgers and enjoy.

EGGPLANT SANDWICH

10 minutes | 25 minutes | 4 Servings

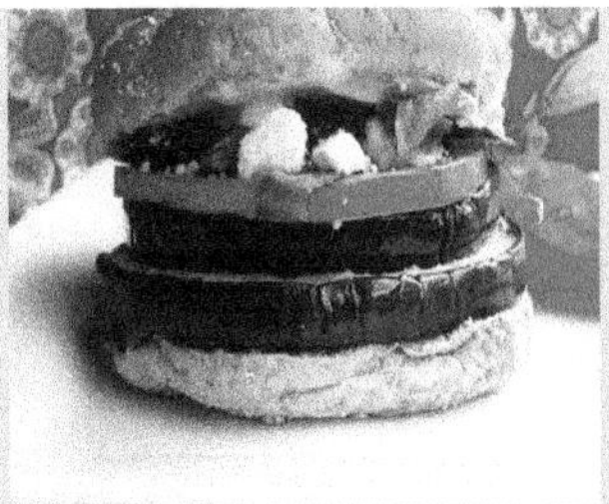

INGREDIENTS

For the Sandwich:

- 2 ciabatta buns
- 1 medium eggplant, peeled, sliced, soaked in salted water
- 1 medium tomato, sliced
- 1/2 of a medium cucumber, sliced
- 1/2 cup arugula
- 4 tablespoons mayo

For the Marinade:

- 1 teaspoon agave syrup

COOKING STEPS

1. Preheat the oven to 350 degrees F.
2. Prepare the marinade and for this, take a small bowl, place all the ingredients in it and whisk until combined.
3. Drain the eggplant slices, pat dry with a kitchen towel, and brush with prepared marinade, arrange them on a baking sheet, and then bake for 20 minutes until done.
4. Assemble the sandwich and for this, slice the bread in half lengthwise, then spread mayonnaise in the bottom half of the bun and top with baked eggplant slices, tomato, and cucumber slices, and sprinkle with salt and black pepper.
5. Top with arugula leaves, cover with the top half of the bun and then cover with aluminum foil.
6. Preheat the grill over a medium-high heat setting and when hot, place prepared sandwiches and grill for 3 to 5 minutes until toasted.
7. Cut each sandwich through the foil into half and serve.

- 1/4 teaspoon salt
- 1/4 teaspoon ground black pepper
- 1 teaspoon smoked paprika
- 1 tablespoon soy sauce
- 1 tablespoon olive oil

Tuna Salad

10 minutes | 0 minutes | 4 Servings

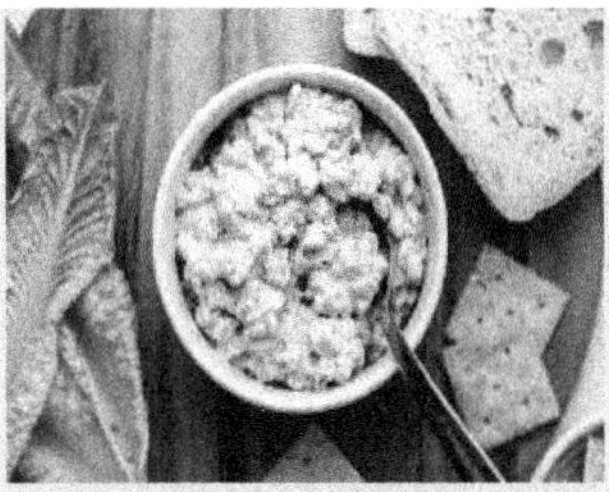

INGREDIENTS

- 1/2 cup chopped celery
- 3 cups cooked chickpeas
- 1 tablespoon capers, chopped
- 2 tablespoons sweet pickle relish
- 1 tablespoon yellow mustard paste
- 2 tablespoons mayonnaise

COOKING STEPS

1. Take a medium bowl, place chickpeas in it, add mustard and mayonnaise, and mash by using a fork until peas are broken.
2. Add remaining ingredients, then stir until well combined.
3. Serve straight away.

FETTUCCINE ALFREDO

10 minutes | 10 minutes | 2 Servings

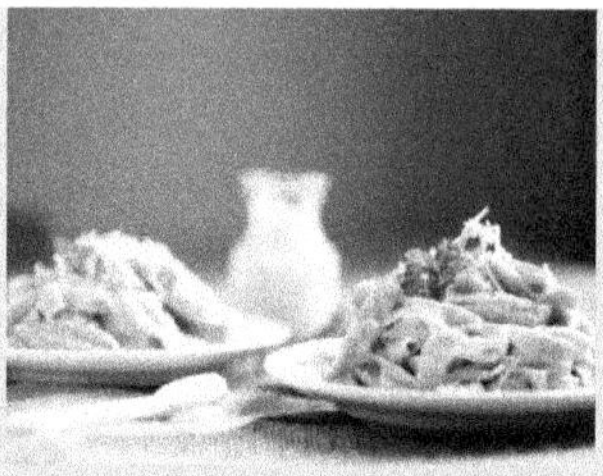

INGREDIENTS

For the sauce:

- 1 cup unsalted cashews (cashews)
- 1 clove garlic
- 2 tablespoons nutritional yeast
- 1 ¼ cups of purified water
- ½ teaspoon salt (adjust to taste)
- 2 tablespoons of parsley
- ½ tablespoon lemon juice

For service:

- Fettuccine Pasta

COOKING STEPS

1. Add the cashew nuts to soak in purified water (Activate) for 8 hours in refrigeration if you live in a warm climate.
2. Once your nuts are soaked you will notice that they have grown in size and their texture is smooth. Drain the water and rinse well.
3. Add all the marked ingredients for the sauce in a blender and blend until you get a homogeneous mixture.
4. Prepare the fettuccine pasta according to the instructions on the package.
5. When your pasta is done, drain. Add in a pot over low heat the sauce that you prepared in the blender.
6. Cook for 2 minutes and add the pasta already cooked. If you like, you can add spinach or chard to your sauce at this point. Cook for 3 more minutes.
7. Serve with fresh parsley.

- Parsley to taste
- Spinach

Lemon, Basil and Orzo Salad

10 minutes

0 minutes

4 Servings

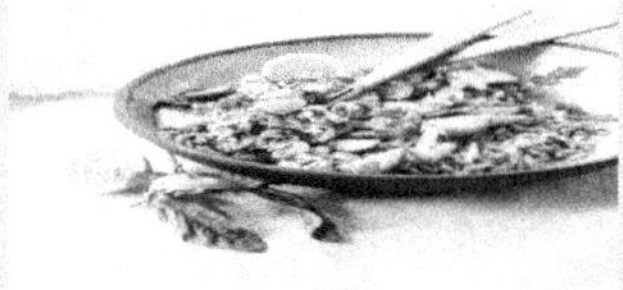

INGREDIENTS

For the Salad:

- 1 cup orzo pasta, cooked
- 2 cup sliced cucumbers
- 1 cup cherry tomatoes, halved
- 1 cup baby arugula

For the Dressing:

- 2 cloves of garlic, peeled
- 1 lemon, zested
- 1 cup basil
- 1/3 cup olive oil
- ¼ teaspoon ground black pepper

COOKING STEPS

1. Prepare the dressing, and for this, place all of its ingredients in a food processor and pulse until smooth.
2. Take a large bowl, place orzo pasta in it, add prepared dressing in it, toss until mixed, then add remaining ingredients for the salad in it and toss until just mixed.
3. Serve straight away

- ½ teaspoon salt
- 2 tablespoons lemon juice

VEGAN CARROTS AND BROCCOLI

10 minutes | 5 minutes | 6 Servings

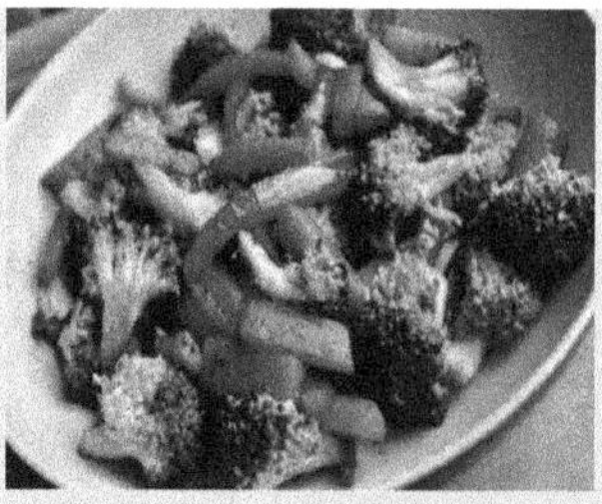

INGREDIENTS

- 4 cups broccoli florets
- 2 carrots, peeled and sliced
- 1/4 cup water
- 1/2 lemon juice
- 1 tsp garlic, minced
- 1 tbsp olive oil
- 1/4 cup vegetable stock
- 1/4 tsp Italian seasoning Salt

COOKING STEPS

1. Add oil into the inner pot of the instant pot and set the pot on sauté mode. Add garlic and sauté for 30 seconds. Add carrots and broccoli and cook for 2 minutes.
2. Add remaining ingredients and stir everything well. Seal pot with lid and cook on high for 3 minutes. Once done, release pressure using quick release.
3. Remove lid. Stir well and serve.

Crunchy Grilled Potatoes with Crispy Sesame

10 minutes

40 minutes

4 Servings

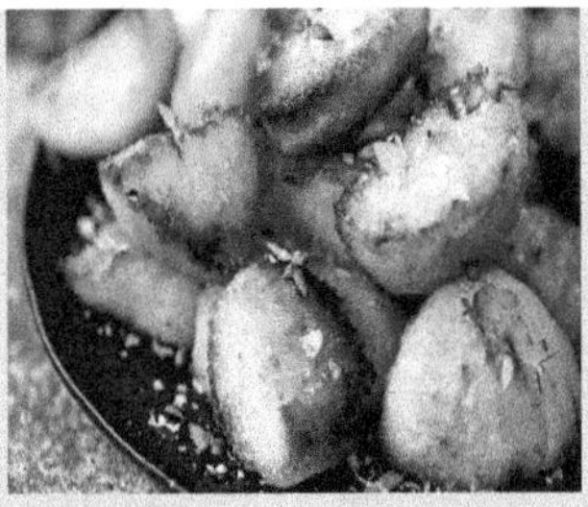

INGREDIENTS

- 8 large potatoes
- 10 grams of olive oil
- 10 grams of sesame seeds
- 1 large clove of garlic

COOKING STEPS

1. Rinse the potatoes together with their skin under cold running water and then pat dry with a kitchen towel.
2. Now cut the potatoes in half with a sharp knife together with the skin.
3. Put the sesame seeds on a plate and distribute them on it.
4. Brush the cut surfaces of the potatoes with the olive oil before placing them on the plate with the sesame seeds so that the sesame seeds stick to the potato half. Repeat the process with all the potato halves.
5. Remove the peel from the garlic clove and cut into fine slices with a sharp knife. Now distribute the slices evenly on the potato halves and press onto them. Squeeze two potato halves together and enclose the garlic in them. To keep them closed, they are wrapped in aluminum foil and baked on the direct embers for about 40 minutes.

TORTILLAS

10 minutes | 10 minutes | 4 Servings

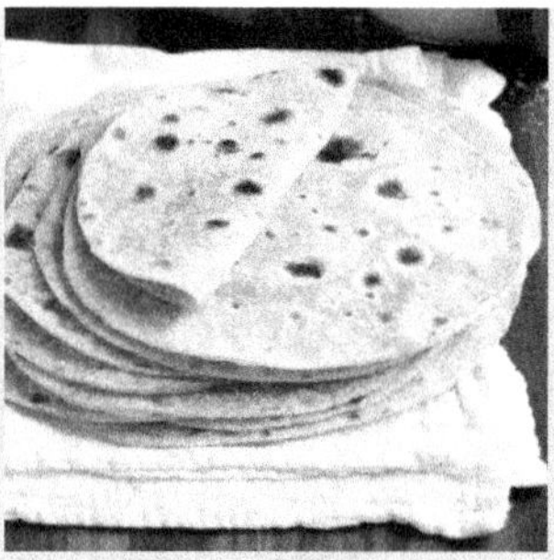

INGREDIENTS

- 250 g wheat flour
- 250 ml of boiling water
- ½ teaspoon salt
- 50 g flour to roll out
- 1 teaspoon of baking powder

COOKING STEPS

1. Put the flour and salt in a bowl, then make a well in the middle.
2. Pour in the boiling water while stirring constantly. Knead the hot dough.
3. Flour the work surface a little and divide the dough into six portions and roll out into tortilla cakes.
4. Fry in a non-oiled pan for one minute on each side.

Almond Bread

10 minutes | 55 minutes | 4 Servings

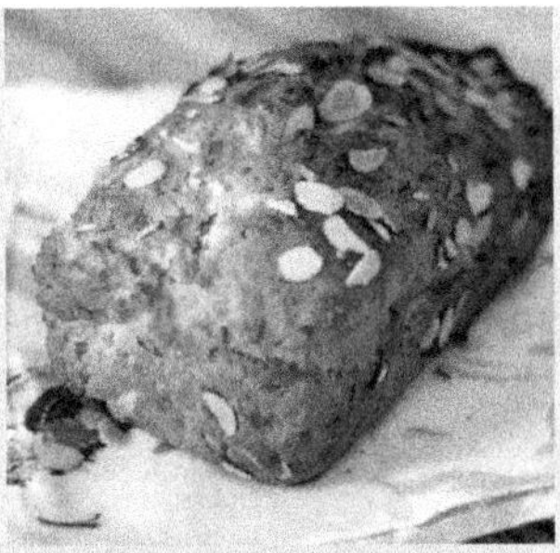

INGREDIENTS

- 400 g of flour
- 150 g whole almonds
- 150 g of tender oat flakes
- 450 ml almond drink (without sugar)
- 1 packet of dry yeast
- 70 g sugar (if you use sweetened almond milk, less sugar)
- 3 tbsp amaretto

COOKING STEPS

1. Roast the almonds in a pan without fat and let them cool. Knead all ingredients into a dough in a food processor.
2. Place the bread dough in a loaf tin lined with baking paper, smooth it out and let it rest for an hour.
3. Bake in a non-preheated oven at 200 ° C top/bottom heat for 55 minutes.
4. Let the almond bread cool on a wire rack.

Braised Pumpkin with Colored Couscous

10 minutes

35 minutes

2 Servings

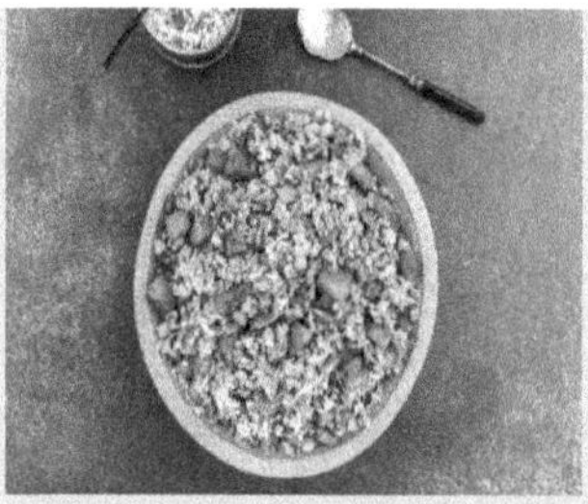

Ingredients

- 500 g pumpkin (Hokkaido, weight without the seeds or the shell)
- 100 g couscous, instant
- 200 ml vegetable stock, vegan
- 3 tablespoons of olive oil
- 250 g tomatoes
- 1 to 2 cloves of garlic
- The freshly squeezed juice of a lemon

Cooking Steps

1. The oven is first preheated to 180 degrees. Then cut the pumpkin into 2 cm thick wedges and place in a baking dish along with chopped garlic, sage leaves, salt, pepper, and chili.
2. Now half of the olive oil is mixed with half of the lemon juice. Spread the mixture evenly over the pumpkin wedges and let them cook in the oven for 30 minutes.
3. In the meantime, bring the vegetable stock to the boil, sprinkle with the couscous, remove from the heat and let it soak.
4. Mix the remaining oil, lemon juice, salt, and pepper with the couscous. Then finely chop the parsley, dice the tomatoes and fold in both.
5. Serve the braised pumpkin with the couscous and sprinkle with fresh parsley if desired.

- Each ½ bunch of fresh parsley and sage
- Salt, pepper, chili flakes

Meatballs with Hunter Sauce

10 minutes | 30 minutes | 2 Servings

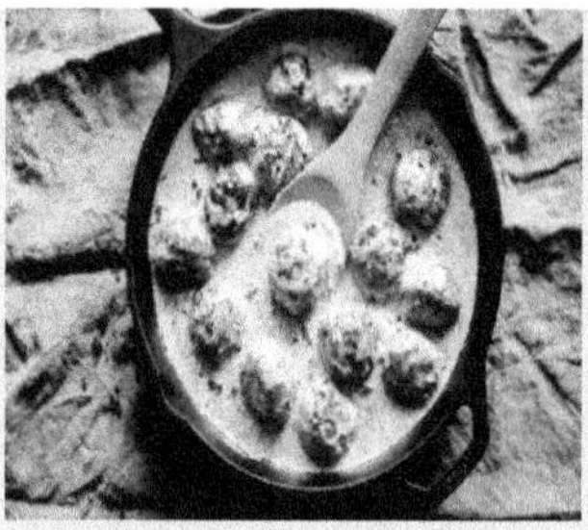

INGREDIENTS

- 250 g mushrooms
- 250 g vegan minced meat
- 1 tbsp flour
- 1 can of coconut milk
- 2 cloves of garlic
- 2 medium onions
- Vegan soy sauce to taste
- 4 tablespoons of olive oil
- Salt, pepper, curry, mustard
- 2 tbsp parsley

COOKING STEPS

1. Cut the onion and garlic into small cubes and divide them in two.
2. Mix the vegan minced meat with onions, garlic, and a little mustard. Then season with salt and pepper. Shape the mince mixture into cakes, bread with flour, and bake in the pan.
3. Clean the mushrooms and cut them into slices. Sauté half of the onions and garlic until translucent, then add the mushrooms and fry them.
4. Deglaze with the coconut milk and let it boil down until the sauce has the desired consistency. Season with soy sauce.
5. Tip: The hunter's sauce also goes well with a seitan steak, for example.

Tofu Spinach Pan with Pine Nuts

15 minutes | 30 minutes | 2 Servings

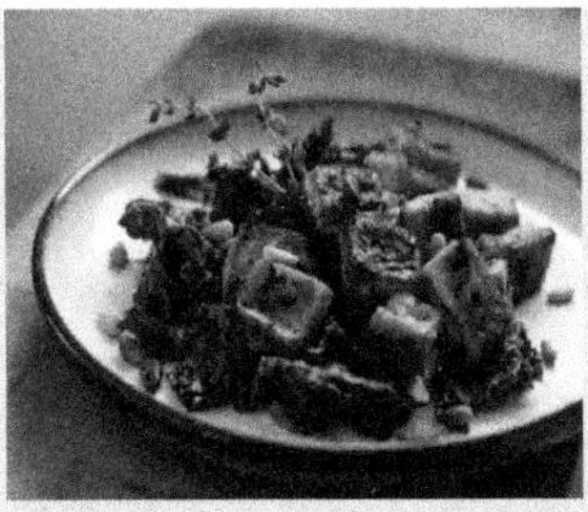

Ingredients

- 400 g natural tofu
- 300 g of fresh baby spinach
- 70 g pine nuts
- 2 shallots
- 2 cloves of garlic
- salt and pepper
- vegetable oil

Cooking Steps

1. First, wring out the tofu thoroughly and cut it into cubes.
2. Wash and clean baby spinach thoroughly.
3. Then put the pine nuts in a pan, roast them until golden brown, and set aside.
4. Now peel the shallots, cut in half, and cut into fine strips. Peel the garlic and cut it into thin slices.
5. Heat a little oil in another, larger pan. Fry the garlic and shallots. Then add tofu, season well, and fry until golden brown.
6. Then add the spinach, mix thoroughly and fry for another 20 minutes over medium heat.
7. Finally fold in the pine nuts, season to taste, and serve with the mentioned side dishes as desired.

STUFFED EGGPLANT WITH TOMATOES AND BASIL

20 minutes

30 minutes

2 Servings

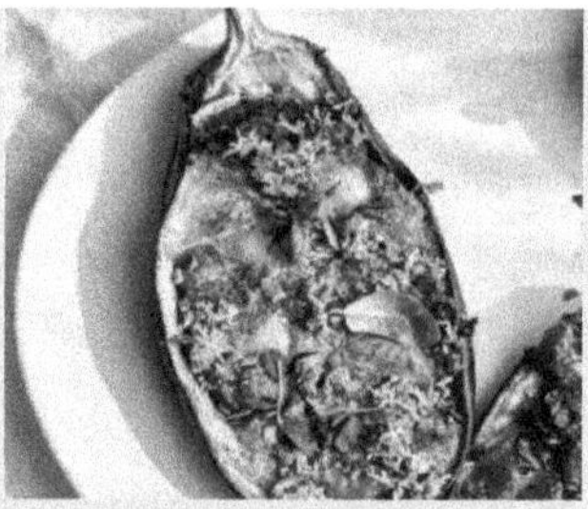

INGREDIENTS

- 2 large eggplants
- 10 cherry tomatoes
- 1 bunch of basil
- 5 tablespoons of olive oil
- 2 teaspoons of dried rosemary
- salt and pepper

COOKING STEPS

1. First, preheat the oven to 180 degrees.
2. Halve the aubergine lengthways, prick several times with a fork, and drizzle with olive oil. Then place on a baking sheet and bake for 30 minutes.
3. In the meantime, wash the cherry tomatoes, remove them from the stalk, and cut them in half.
4. Wash the basil and pat dry.
5. Take the aubergines out of the oven and spoon out the insides with a spoon.
6. Then spread the tomatoes and basil on top, season with rosemary, and bake for 15 minutes.
7. Arrange at the end and serve with some bread.

Cheesy Macaroni with Broccoli

10 minutes | 25 minutes | 6 Servings

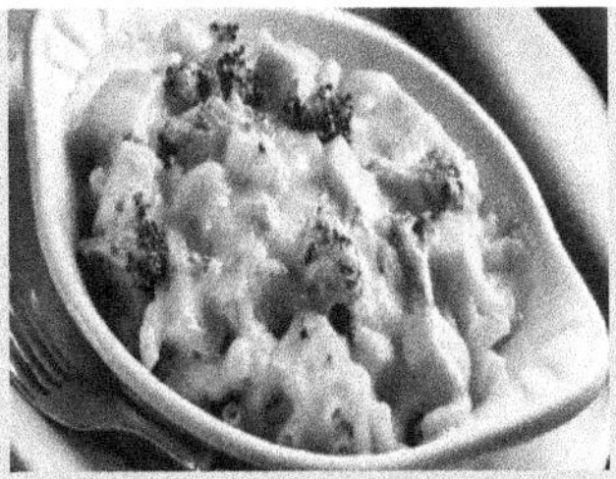

Ingredients

- 1/3 cup melted coconut oil
- ¼ cup nutritional yeast
- 1 tablespoon tomato paste
- 1 tablespoon dried mustard
- 2 garlic cloves, minced
- 1 ½ teaspoons salt
- ½ teaspoon ground turmeric
- 4 ½ cups almond milk
- 3 cups cauliflower florets, chopped

Cooking Steps

1. Place a suitably sized saucepan over medium heat and add coconut oil.
2. Stir in mustard, yeast, garlic, salt, tomato paste, and turmeric.
3. Cook for 1 minute then add almond milk, cashews, and cauliflower florets.
4. Cook for 20 minutes on a simmer.
5. Transfer the cauliflower mixture to a blender jug then blend until smooth.
6. Stir in vinegar and blend until creamy.
7. Fill a suitably-sized pot with salted water and bring it to a boil on high heat.
8. Add pasta to the boiling water.
9. Place a steamer basket over the boiling water and add broccoli to the basket.
10. Cook until the pasta is al dente. Drain and rinse the pasta and transfer the broccoli to a bowl.
11. Add the cooked pasta to the cauliflower-cashews sauce.
12. Toss in broccoli florets, salt, and black pepper.

- 1 cup raw cashews, chopped
- 1 lb. shell pasta
- 1 tablespoon white vinegar
- 3 cups broccoli florets

13. Mix well then serve.

Pumpkin Risotto

5 minutes

20 minutes

4 Servings

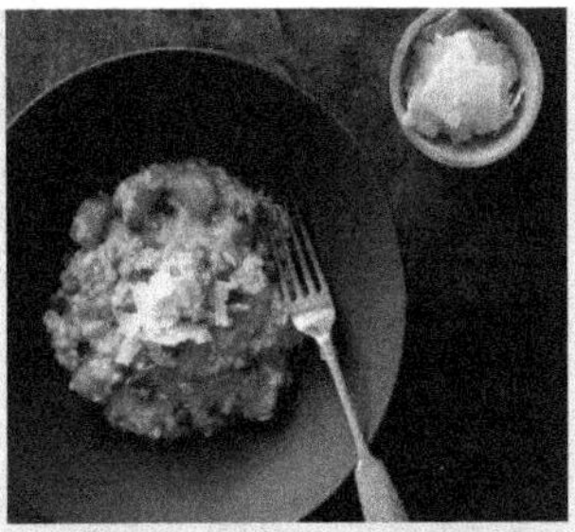

INGREDIENTS

- 1 cup Arborio rice
- ½ cup cooked and chopped pumpkin
- 1/2 cup mushrooms
- 1 rib of celery, diced
- ½ of a medium white onion, peeled, diced
- ½ teaspoon minced garlic
- ½ teaspoon salt
- 1/3 teaspoon ground black pepper
- 1 tablespoon olive oil

COOKING STEPS

1. Take a medium saucepan, place it over medium heat, add oil and when hot, add onion and celery, stir in garlic and cook for 3 minutes until onions begin to soften.
2. Add mushrooms, season with salt and black pepper, and cook for 5 minutes.
3. Add rice, pour in pumpkin puree, then gradually pour in the stock until rice soaked up all the liquid and have turned soft.
4. Add butter, remove the pan from heat, stir until creamy mixture comes together, and then serve.

- ½ tablespoon coconut butter
- 1 cup pumpkin puree
- 2 cups vegetable stock

VEGETABLE MANCHEGO GAZPACHO

10 minutes | 30 minutes | 2 Servings

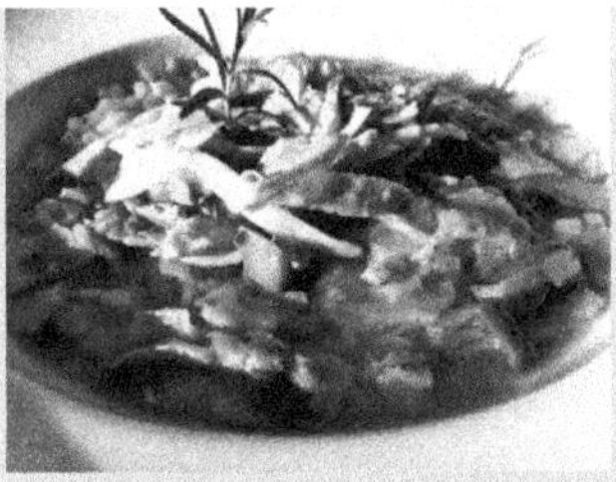

INGREDIENTS

- 3 tablespoons of extra virgin olive oil
- 1 red bell pepper
- 1 white or purple onion
- 2 cloves of garlic
- 4 or 5 artichokes
- 1 tomato, peeled and grated
- 300 g of ashen cakes for gazpacho
- Water
- Juice of half an orange
- Salt

COOKING STEPS

1. Cook the artichokes.
2. We start by removing the hard leaves of the artichokes, cutting the tips, and peeling the stem. Then we cook them in salted water and the juice of half an orange. When they are tender, we remove them from the heat and reserve them. We will reserve the cooking water as well, as we will use it as a broth to cook our vegetable gazpacho manchego.
3. Prepare the sauté.
4. In a large casserole or frying pan, we heat the extra virgin olive oil and fry the onion and pepper cut into small pieces, and the garlic that we can press so that it is then imperceptible in the stew. Lightly salt and fry over medium-low heat until the vegetables are tender.
5. Add the ashen cakes, stir well and cover the artichokes with the cooking water. We lower the heat just enough to keep a light boil and leave it for about ten minutes. If we see that it is too dry, add a little more broth or, if we don't have it, water with a pinch of salt.

6. Add the artichokes that we had reserved.

7. Finally, we chop the artichokes that we had reserved and, when there are about 5 minutes to finish cooking, we add them to the stew that we can leave more or less soupy depending on the tastes of each one.

Cavolo Nero and Pea Farro Pilaf

10 minutes	40 minutes	4 Servings

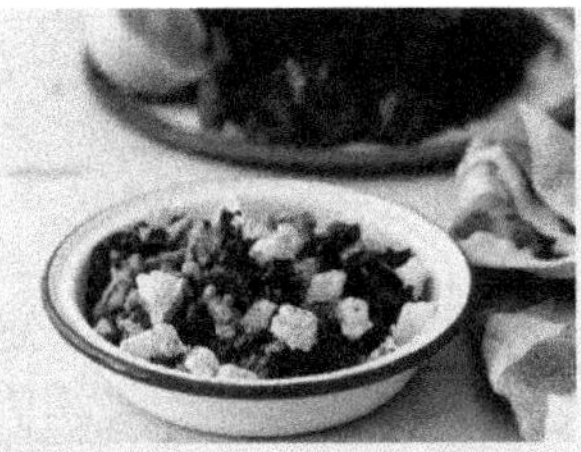

Ingredients

- 1 cup green peas
- 4 cups cavolo nero, torn into pieces
- ½ cup hummus
- ½ cup scallions, sliced
- 1 garlic clove, minced
- 1 cup farro
- 2 cups water
- 1 cup chopped tomatoes
- 1 tbsp tomato paste
- 1 tsp cumin
- ½ tsp oregano

Cooking Steps

1. Heat the olive oil in a skillet over medium heat, then add in scallions, sauté until tender.
2. Add in garlic, cumin, and oregano and cook for another 30 seconds.
3. Stir in farro, water, chopped tomatoes, and tomato paste.
4. Bring to a boil, then lower the heat, then simmer for 30-40 minutes. Stir in peas, cavolo nero, salt, and black pepper.
5. Let sit covered for 8 minutes.
6. Serve topped with hummus and cilantro.

- 2 tbsp fresh cilantro, chopped
- 2 tbsp olive oil
- Salt and black pepper to taste

Feta and Chard Couscous

10 minutes	10 minutes	4 Servings

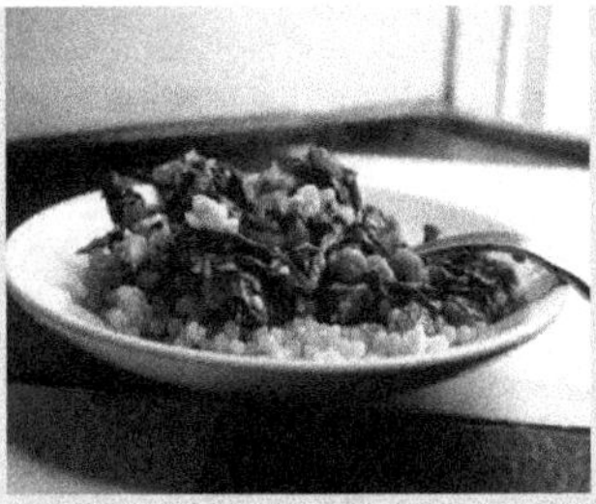

Ingredients

- 2 tbsp olive oil
- 10 oz couscous
- 2 garlic cloves, minced
- 1 cup raisins
- ½ cup feta cheese, crumbled
- 1 bunch of Swiss chard, chopped

Cooking Steps

1. In a bowl, place couscous and cover with hot water. Let sit covered for 10 minutes.
2. Using a fork fluff it. Warm the olive oil in a skillet over medium heat and sauté garlic for a minute.
3. Stir in couscous, raisins, and chard. Serve topped with feta cheese.

LEMONY SPROUTS

10 minutes | 10 minutes | 4 Servings

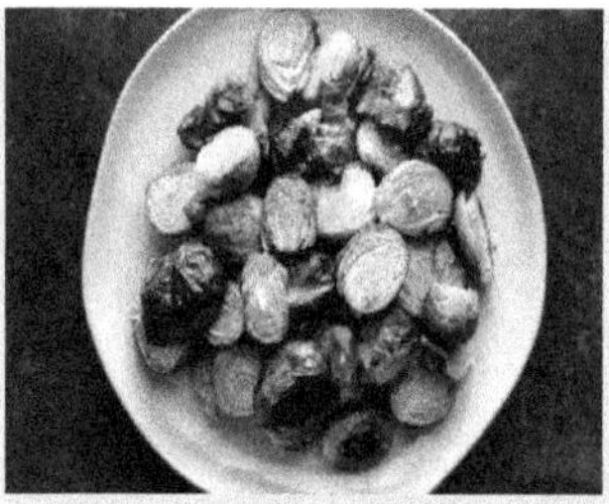

INGREDIENTS

- pound Brussels sprouts, trimmed and shredded
- 8 tablespoons olive oil
- 1 lemon, juice, and zested
- Sunflower seeds and pepper to taste
- ¾ cup spicy almond and seed mix

COOKING STEPS

1. Take a bowl and mix in lemon juice, sunflower seeds, pepper, and olive oil. Mix well.
2. Stir in shredded Brussels sprouts and toss. Let it sit for 10 minutes.
3. Add nuts and toss. Serve and enjoy!

VEGGIES WITH RED LENTILS

10 minutes | 25 minutes | 6 Servings

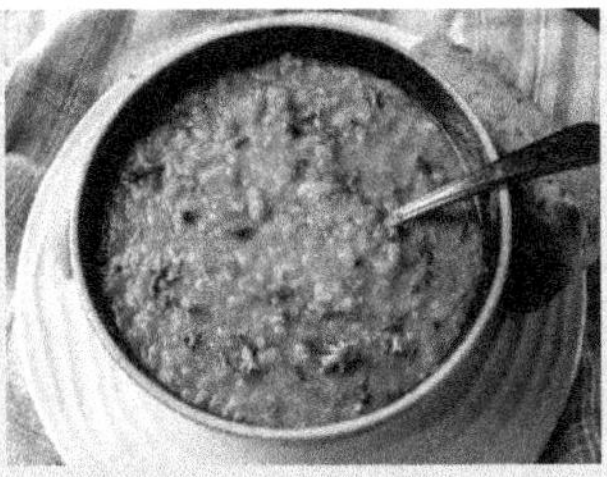

INGREDIENTS

- 2 tablespoons coconut oil
- 12 fresh curry leaves
- 1 teaspoon cumin seeds
- 1 teaspoon brown mustard seeds
- 1 medium onion, chopped finely
- 4 garlic cloves, chopped finely
- 3 tablespoons fresh ginger, minced
- 1 Serrano chile, chopped finely
- 1½ cups red lentils

COOKING STEPS

1. In a sizable pan, melt coconut oil on medium-high heat.
2. Add curry leaves, cumin seeds, and mustard seeds and sauté for around a few seconds.
3. Add onion and sauté for 5 minutes.
4. Add garlic, ginger, and Serrano chile and sauté for approximately half a minute.
5. Add lentils, turmeric, salt, coconut milk, and water and produce to your boil, stirring occasionally.
6. Stir inside the vegetables and again bring to your boil.
7. Reduce heat to low and simmer, covered for around 20-25 minutes or till the desired doneness.
8. Stir in lime juice and garam masala and immediately, remove from heat.
9. Serve hot.

- 1 teaspoon ground turmeric
- Salt, to taste
- 1 (14-ounce) can coconut milk
- 4½ cups water
- 2 cups cauliflower, cut into 1-inch florets
- 2½ cups butternut squash, peeled and cubed
- 1 large Yukon gold potato, peeled and cut into cubes
- 2 tablespoons fresh lime juice
- 1 tablespoon garam masala

Creamy Panna Cotta with Fruity Raspberry Sauce

10 minutes | 10 minutes | 2 Servings

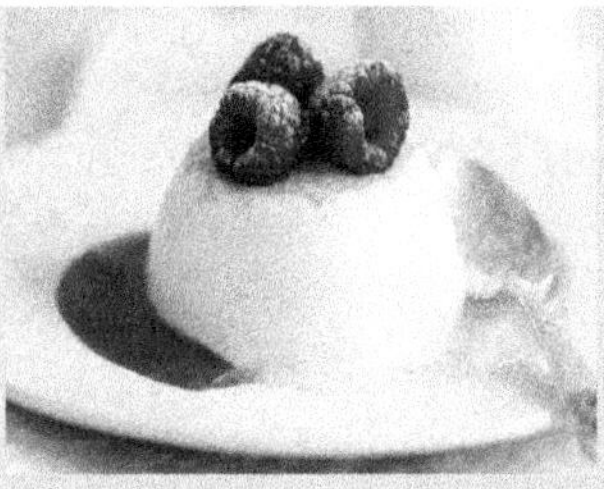

INGREDIENTS

- 200 grams of soy cream
- 3 tbsp agave syrup
- 3 grams of agar agar
- 1 small vanilla pod
- 100 grams of fresh raspberries (Alternatively, raspberries from the freezer can be used)
- some brown sugar as needed

COOKING STEPS

1. The soy cream is put together with the agave syrup in a saucepan and stirred thoroughly in it.
2. When the mass is well mixed, the agar agar can then be added to the pot and stirred well. Now the vanilla pod is cut lengthways so that the pulp can be scraped out of the two halves with the help of a sharp knife.
3. The black pulp of the vanilla is now also added to the pot. Now stir the contents of the pot again well and thoroughly before slowly heating it, stirring constantly. Let the mixture boil for about a minute before removing the pot from the stove. It is important that the mixture inside the pot boils for at least one minute, otherwise the agar agar may not bind properly.
4. After a minute, the saucepan is removed from the stove and the mass is divided between two bowls. Now put the mixture in the refrigerator for at least 4 hours.
5. When the panna cotta is ready, the raspberry sauce can be prepared. Wash the fresh raspberries or thaw the frozen raspberries and puree them with a little brown sugar in a

blender or with the help of a hand blender to a fine sauce. Turn the panna cotta out onto a plate and serve with the raspberry sauce.

Creamy Chocolate Pudding with Avocado and Bananas

10 minutes | 5 minutes | 2 Servings

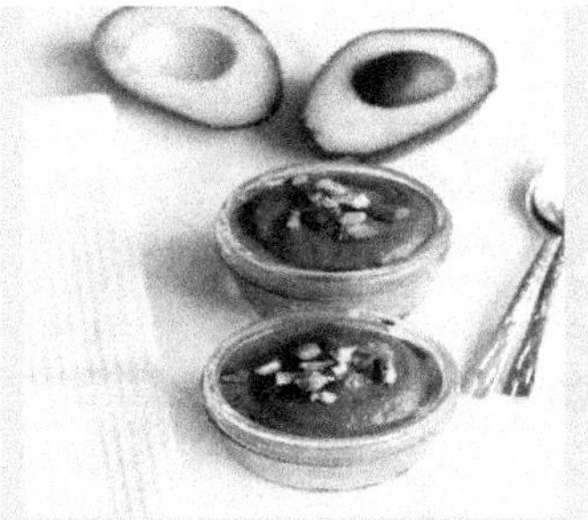

INGREDIENTS

- 2 small bananas
- 1 large ripe and creamy avocado
- 30 grams of unsweetened and de-oiled cocoa powder
- 10 grams of agave syrup

COOKING STEPS

1. Remove the peel from the bananas and mash them into a fine puree in a bowl with the help of a fork.
2. Now halve the avocado lengthways and first remove the stone from the inside of the pulp with the help of a spoon, before the spoon is also used to loosen the pulp from the peel of the avocado.
3. With the help of a knife, the pulp is cut into fine cubes.
4. Put the avocado cubes together with the mashed banana, cocoa powder, and agave syrup in a blender or fill into a tall container so that you can puree it into a fine pudding with the help of a hand blender.
5. The pudding is now divided into two bowls and refrigerated for about 30 minutes before it can be enjoyed.

MANGO-CREAM

15 minutes

0 minutes

4 Servings

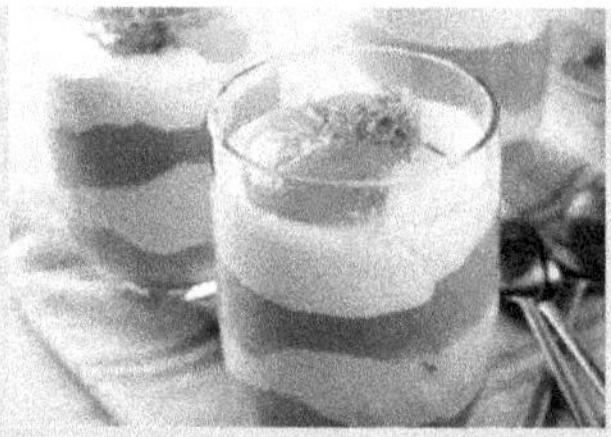

INGREDIENTS

- 1 mango, ripe
- 200 ml coconut milk
- 50 grams of sugar
- 1 tbsp lime juice
- 1 stalk of mint

COOKING STEPS

1. Peel the mango first, cut away the core. Then roughly chop the mango and mix it with sugar, coconut milk, and lime juice. Mix the ingredients together with a blender.
2. Now put the mango cream in a bowl and put it in the fridge for around 2 hours.
3. Garnish with mint before serving.

Caramel Cream

10 minutes | 10 minutes | 2 Servings

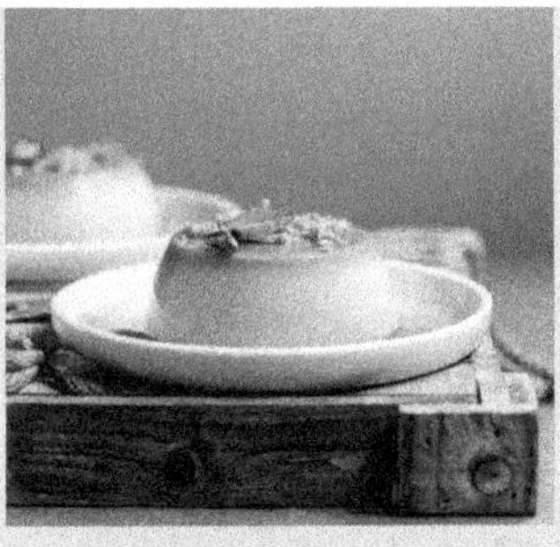

Ingredients

- 400 ml coconut milk
- 100 g of sugar
- ½ teaspoon salt

Cooking Steps

1. Place the ingredients into a saucepan, then bring to the boil.
2. Cook on medium heat for 1 hour, stirring Simmer on medium heat for 1 hour, stirring sporadically.
3. Fill the cream into one or more sterile screw-top jars. Let the caramel cream cool down.

TOFU AND STRAWBERRY MOUSSE

10 minutes | 10 minutes | 2 Servings

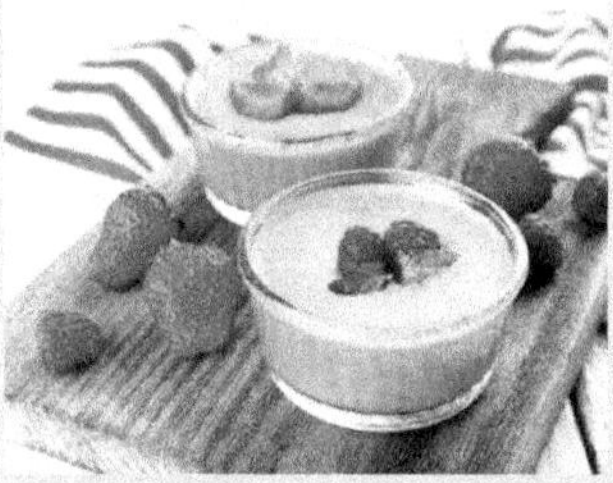

INGREDIENTS

- 200g silky tofu
- 200 g of clean strawberries
- 80/100 g of sugar
- 1 teaspoon cornstarch

COOKING STEPS

1. Blend the strawberries and the resulting puree put them in a saucepan.
2. Add the sugar, the cornstarch, and bring to the fire while mixing so that it does not stick.
3. When the sauce takes consistency, blend the tofu, and mix with the sauce.
4. Place the mousse in cups and refrigerate for at least 3 hours before consuming.

WATERMELON LOLLIES

15 minutes | 0 minutes | 5 Servings

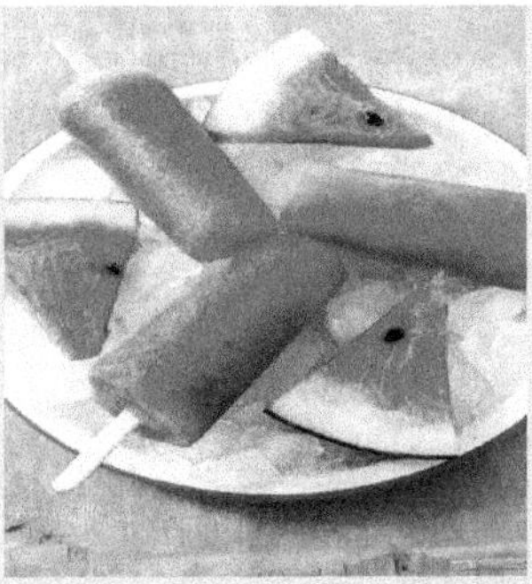

INGREDIENTS

- ½ cup watermelon, cubed
- 2 tablespoons lemon juice, freshly squeezed
- ½ cup water
- 1 tablespoon stevia

COOKING STEPS

1. In a food processor, put cubed watermelon. Process until smooth. Divide an equal amount of the mixture into an ice pop container. Place inside the freezer for 1 hour. Meanwhile, in a small bowl, put together lemon juice, water, and stevia. Mix well. Pour over frozen watermelon lollies.
2. Add in pop sticks. Freeze for another hour. Pry out watermelon lollies.
3. Serve.

RASPBERRY-CHOCO SHAKE

5 minutes

0 minutes

1 Servings

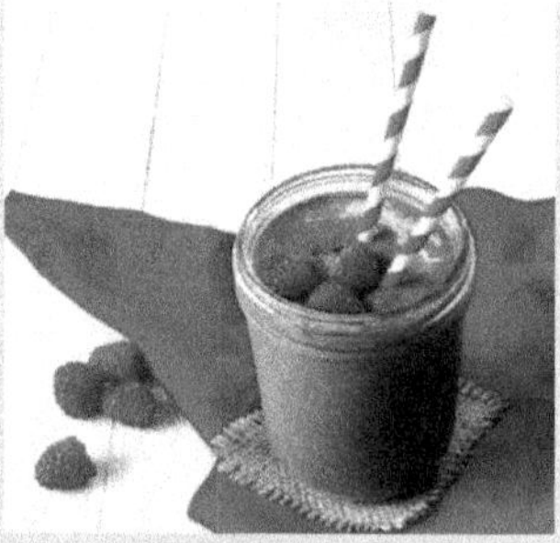

INGREDIENTS

- ¼ cup heavy cream, liquid
- 1 tbsp cocoa powder
- 1 packet Stevia, or more to taste
- ¼ cup raspberries
- 1 ½ cups water

COOKING STEPS

1. Add all the ingredients to a blender. Blend until smooth and creamy.
2. Serve and enjoy.

CPSIA information can be obtained
at www.ICGtesting.com
Printed in the USA
BVHW010735060521
606332BV00023B/417

9 781802 610475